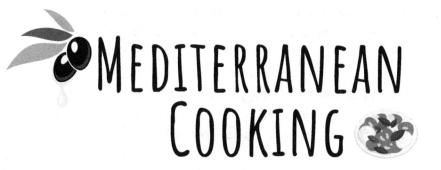 MEDITERRANEAN COOKING

breakfast, lunch, snacks and dinner recipes for your Mediterranean Diet

Natalia Melania Rivera

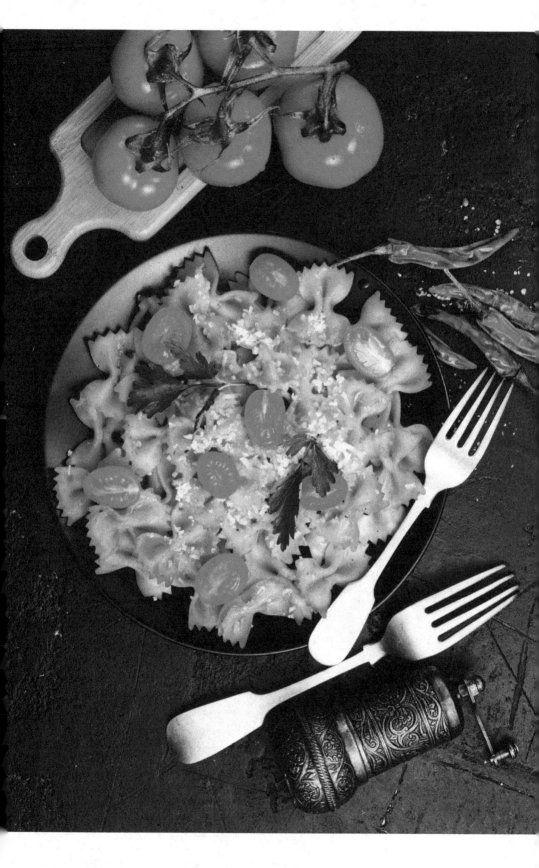

Table of Contents

Table of Contents

Dinner

Breakfast

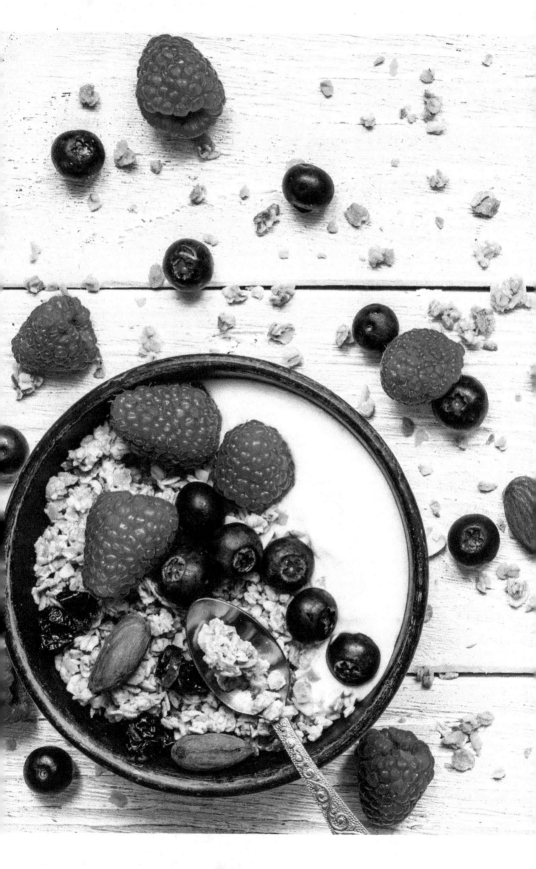

1. Watermelon Smoothie

PREPARATION: 5 MIN   **COOKING:** 0 MIN   **SERVES:** 2

Ingredients

- 2 slices of watermelon
- 1 juice lyme

Directions

1 Blend everything and garnish with lyme

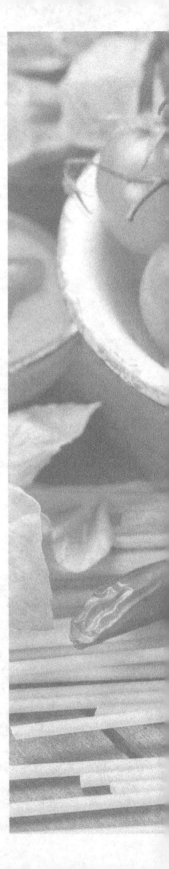

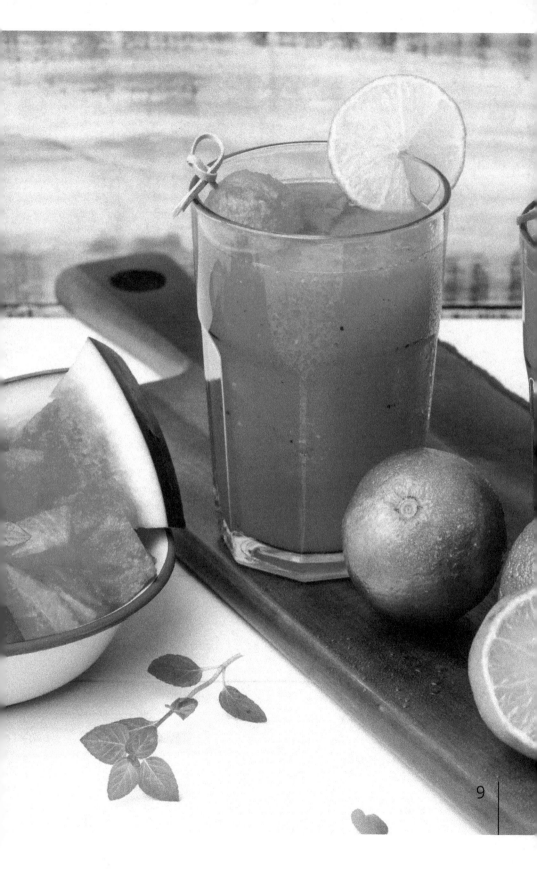

2. Green-Yellow Toast

PREPARATION: 5 MIN

COOKING: 5 MIN

SERVES: 1

Ingredients

- 2 slices of whole-grain bread
- ½ avocado
- 1 egg
- Pinch of pink salt and pepper

Directions

1. First of all, cook a scrambled egg with a pinch of salt and pepper. Meanwhile, toast the bread slices.

2. When the toasted bread is ready, spreading avocado on it and then the scrambled egg.

3. Serve and enjoy the breakfast!

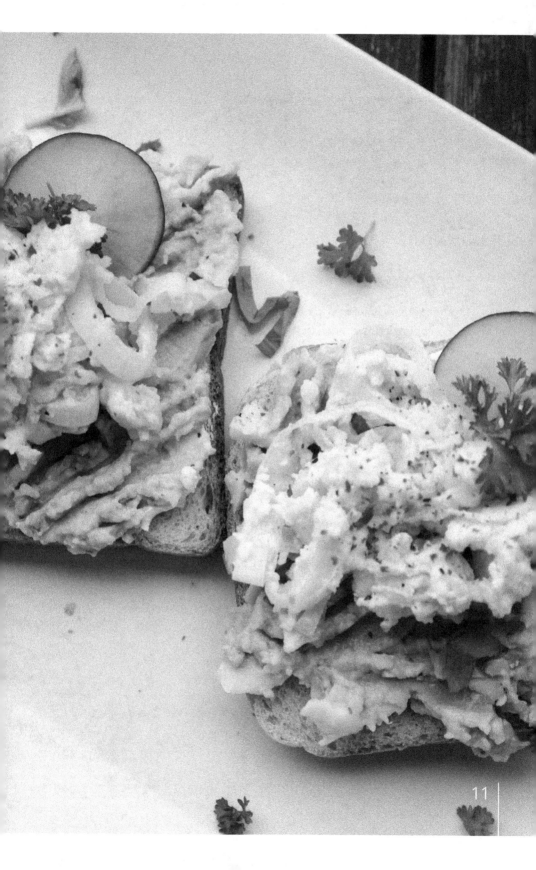

3. Cocoa Pancakes

PREPARATION: 5 MIN

COOKING: 6 MIN

SERVES: 2

Ingredients

- 1 teaspoon vanilla extract
- 2 tablespoons almond butter
- 3 tablespoons cocoa powder
- 2 eggs
- ½ cup of milk
- 2 tablespoons of flour

Directions

1 Turn on a skillet on medium-low heat and grease it with butter. In a blender, put all ingredients and pulse until smooth.

2 Pour ¼ cup batter into the skillet and form a pancake. Cook for 3 minutes on each side.

3 Serve and Enjoy!

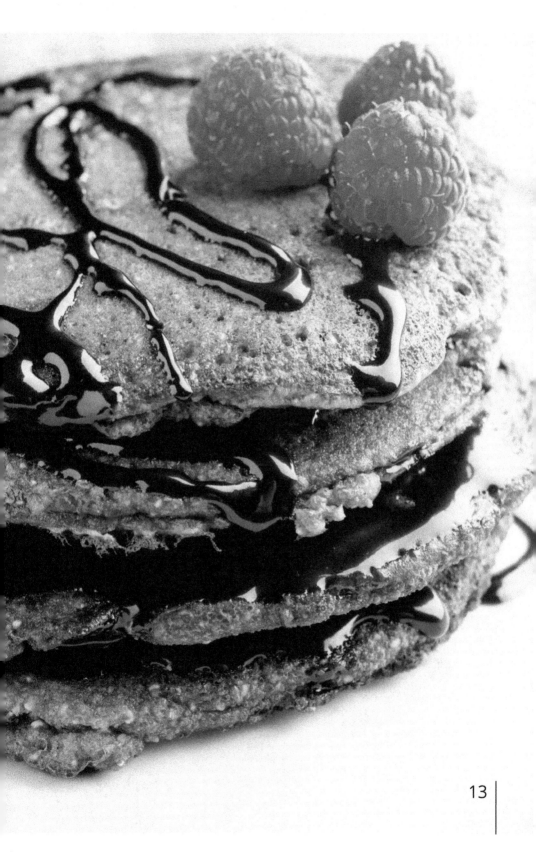

4. Honey Sesam Bars

PREPARATION: 6-7 MIN   COOKING: 30 MIN   SERVES: 10-12 portions

Ingredients

- 180 g sesame seeds
- 180 g honey
- 1 tablespoon of lemon zest

Directions

1 Turn on a skillet on heat and add the sesame seeds and toast them for 3 minutes until golden.

2 Add the honey and wait for it to come to a boil with a wooden spoon constantly mixing. Simmer for 5 minutes.

3 Turn off the skillet and add the lemon zest. Cool for 20 minutes. Now you can serve!

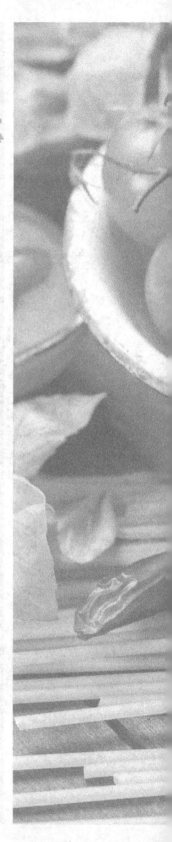

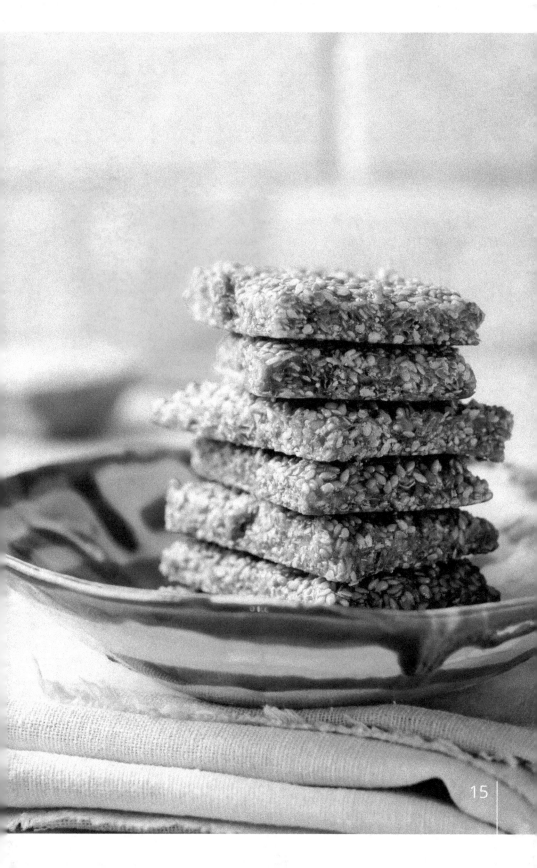

5. Almond Biscuits

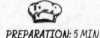
PREPARATION: 5 MIN

COOKING: 6-7 MIN

SERVES: 1

Ingredients

- 2 cups of almond meal
- 2 cups of caster sugar
- 3 eggs
- Grated rind of an orange
- Icing sugar for garnish

Directions

1 In a bowl, mix the almond meal with caster sugar and grated zest of an orange.

2 Add three eggs and mix. Shape the mixture into balls about the size of a walnut and place them on a baking tray. Cook for 15 minutes.

3 Serve cool with icing sugar.

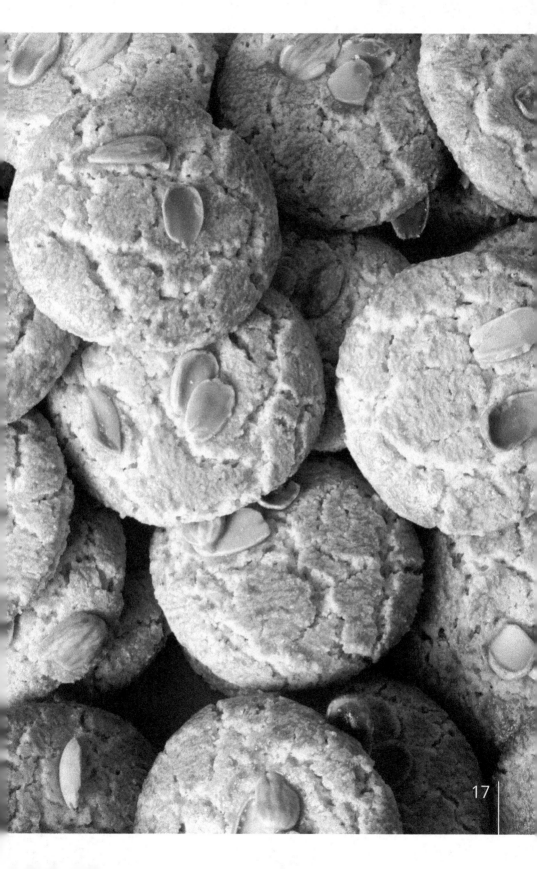

6. Greek Fruit-Cereal Mix

PREPARATION: 5 MIN

COOKING: 0 MIN

SERVES: 2

Ingredients

- 1 cup of Greek yogurt
- ½ cup of cereal mix
- 1 tablespoon of raspberries
- 2 sliced figs

Directions

1. In a small bowl, add the Greek Yoghurt, cereal mix, raspberries, and sliced figs.

2. Serve and enjoy the breakfast!

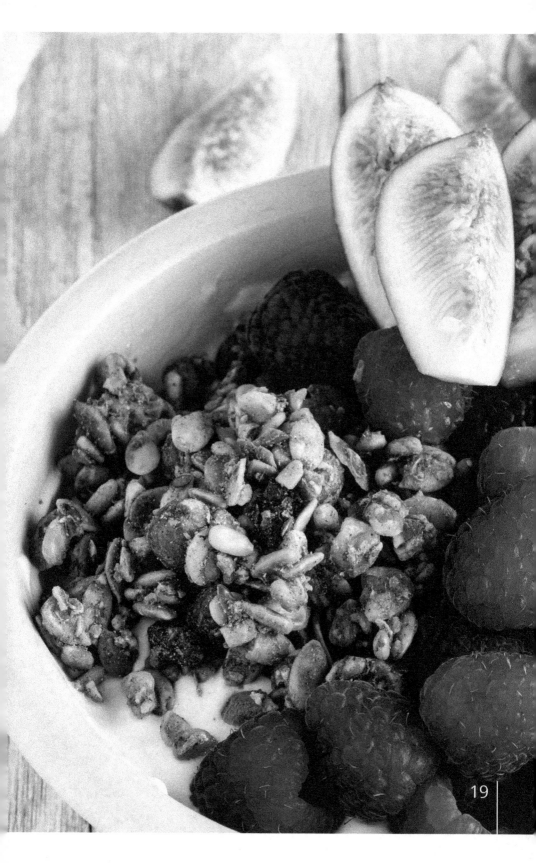

7.Mousse Greek Yogurt

PREPARATION: 5 MIN

COOKING: 0 MIN

SERVES: 4

Ingredients

- 50 g of icing sugar
- 250 g of Greek yogurt
- 200 g of whip cream

Directions

1 In a bowl, put all ingredients and mix all with the electric mixer.

2 Fill with four glass cup and Serve with fruits!

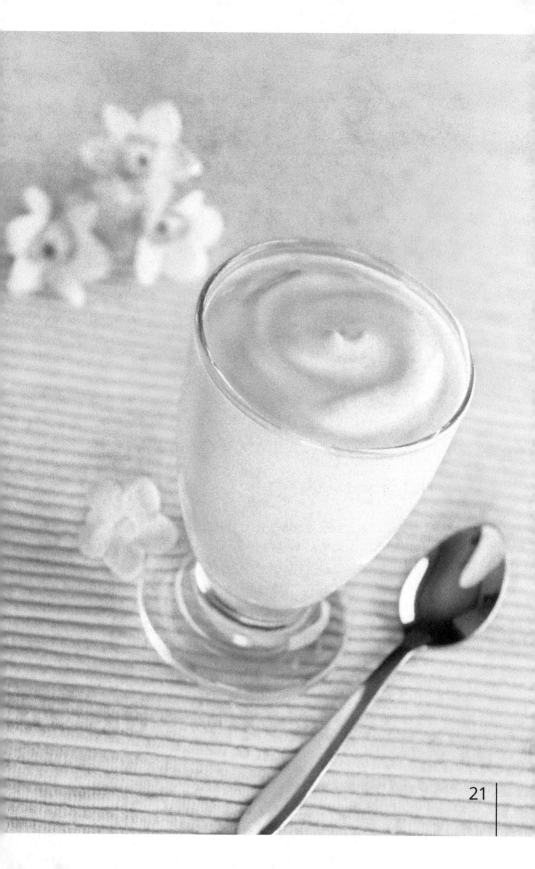

8. Orange Granita

PREPARATION: 20 MIN   **COOKING:** 2 hours   **SERVES:** 6

Ingredients

- 300 ml of orange juice
- 500 ml of water
- 200 g of sugar

Directions

1 First of all, dissolve 200 g of sugar in 500 ml of water in a pot. Then turn off the pot. When the syrup is cold, add the orange juice and mix.

2 Now put the syrup into a small casserole and freeze it for 30 minutes.
After 30 minutes, take the casserole and chopped the ice syrup. Freeze all again for 1 1/2 hours.

3 Take the ice syrup and mix it into the mixer.
Distribute the granita into six cups and serve!

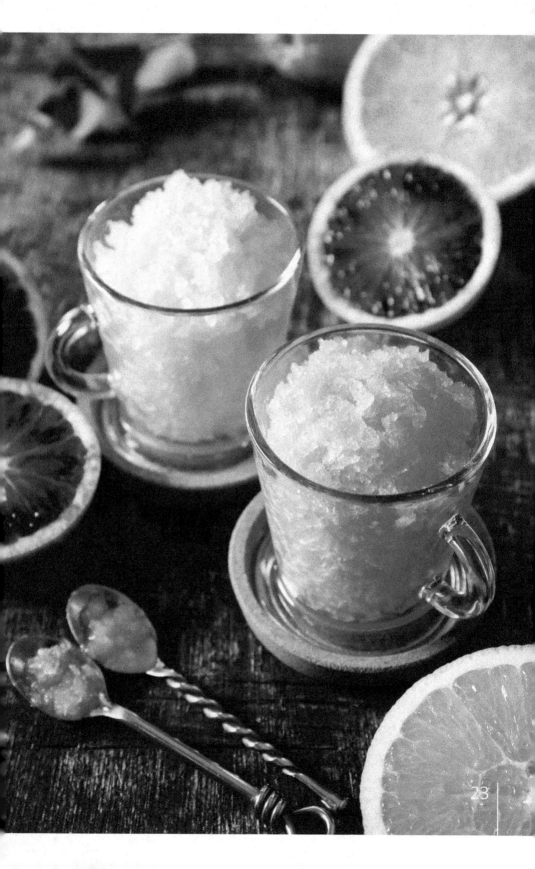

9. Savory Rosemary Italian Cookies

PREPARATION : 8 MIN

COOKING: 6 MIN

SERVES:4

Ingredients

- 1 cup flour
- 3 teaspoons fresh rosemary chopped
- ½ teaspoons salt
- 4 tablespoons Parmesan cheese
- 4 tablespoons butter, softened

Directions

1 In a bowl, mix flour, rosemary, salt, Parmesan cheese, butter until the mixture pulls away from the sides of the bowl.

2 In parchment paper, place the mixture and knead it again. Make mini balls and freeze for 30 minutes. Preheat the oven to 350°F.

3 After 30 minutes, place the balls in a baking pan and bake for 30 minutes until golden brown.
Serve and Enjoy!

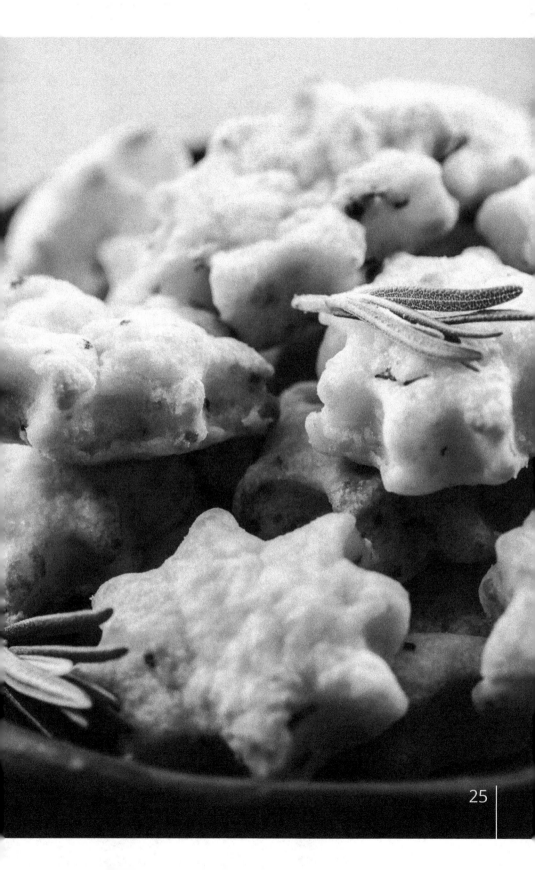

10. Vegetable eggs mini pie oven

PREPARATION: 8 MIN

COOKING: 20 MIN

SERVES: 4

Ingredients

- 6 cherry tomatoes chopped
- 1 small eggplant chopped
- 1 red pepper chopped
- 1 potato chopped
- 1 onion chopped
- 4 teaspoons parsley
- 4 eggs
- Salt
- Pepper
- 2 tablespoons Parmesan cheese

Directions

1 Preheat your oven to 350°F In a bowl, whisk eggs with salt and pepper. Then add all vegetables and Parmesan cheese and mix with a wooden spoon.

2 Pour the mixture into cookie cups.
Bake for 20 minutes to 350°F.

3 Serve and Enjoy!

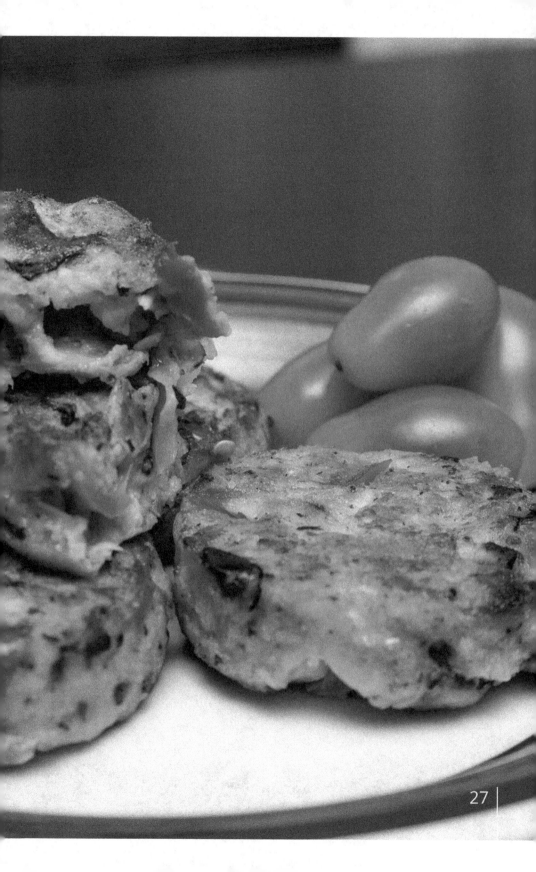

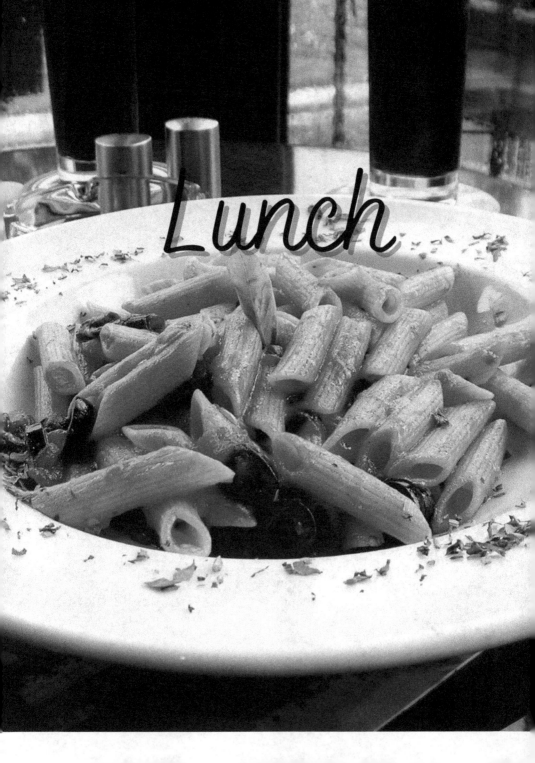

Lunch

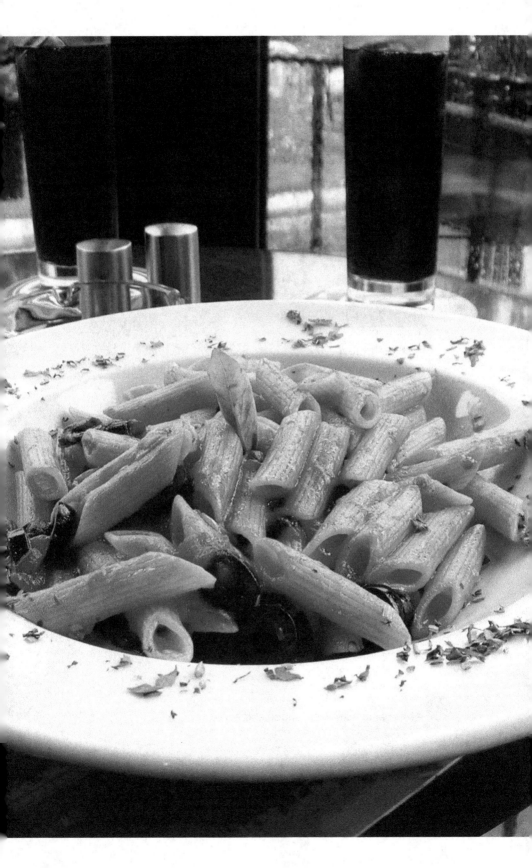

11. Sicilian Tomato Basil Pasta

 PREPARATION: 5 MIN   COOKING: 25 MIN   SERVES: 2

Ingredients

- 200 g of dry spaghetti pasta
- ¾ tomato puree
- 1 ½ of garlic clove
- 2 tablespoons of virgin olive oil
- 1 teaspoon of salt
- 7 basil leaves

Directions

1 Pasta sauce
In a skillet, sauté the garlic cloves with virgin olive oil for 4 minutes, then add tomato puree and basil and cook for 15 minutes.

2 Meanwhile, cook the pasta: take the pot and fill with water and bring it to a boil. Pour the salt into the boiling water. When the salt is dissolved, put the pasta and cook as instructed.

3 Mix pasta with pasta sauce and serve.

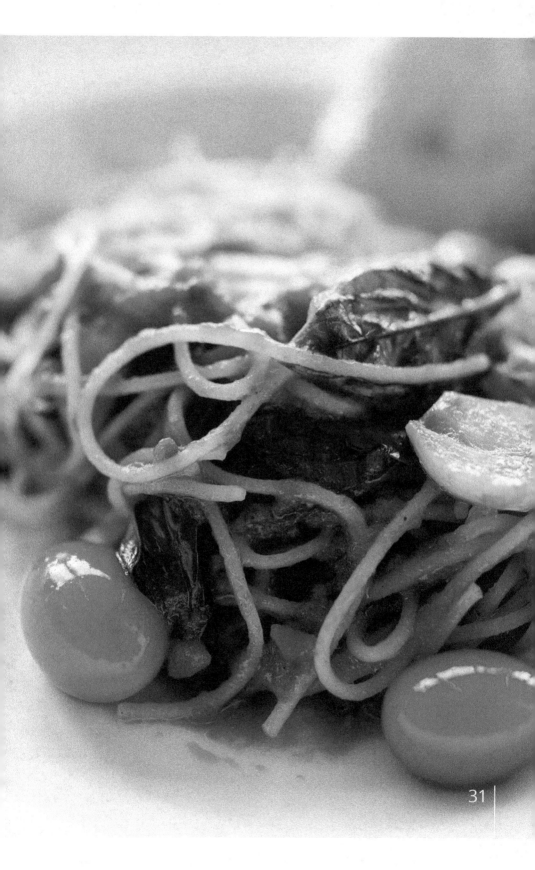

12. Pan-Fried Fillets of Codfish

PREPARATION: 5 MIN

COOKING: 20 MIN

SERVES: 2

Ingredients

- 2 codfish fillets
- 1 courgette, sliced
- 2 teaspoons of lemon juice
- 2 tablespoons of olive oil
- ½ teaspoon of salt
- 7 cherry tomatoes, sliced
- 2 tablespoons of black olives
- 1 teaspoon of rosemary

Directions

1. In a pan, add olive oil and codfish fillets, salt. Then add the courgette, lemon juice, cherry tomatoes, black olives, rosemary and cover the pan.

2. Cook for 20 minutes on medium heat. Serve and enjoy!

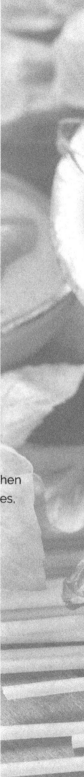

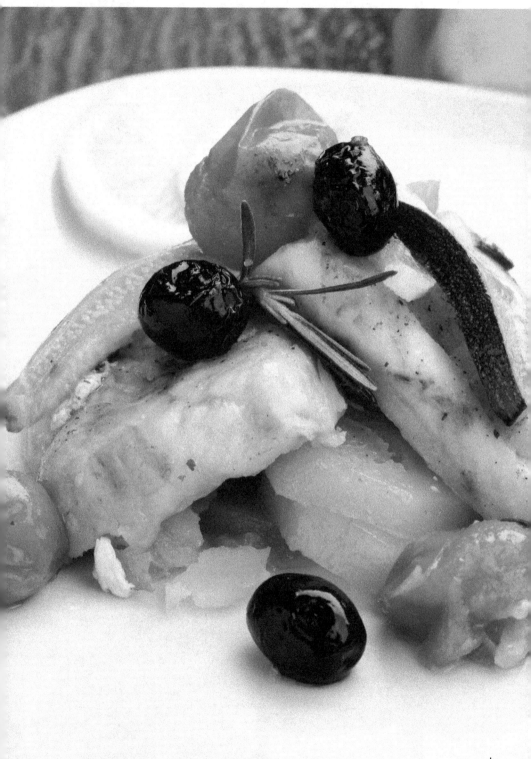

13. Halibut Steaks Baked Marinated

PREPARATION: 20 MIN

COOKING: 30 MIN

SERVES: 2

Ingredients

- 2 halibut steaks
- 2 teaspoons of lemon juice
- 2 tablespoons of olive oil
- 1 teaspoon of salt
- 1 teaspoon of pepper
- 1 teaspoon of thyme
- 1 teaspoon of rosemary

Directions

1 In a casserole, put the olive oil, lemon juice, garlic powder and all spices.

2 Place halibut steaks and rub the seasonings. Put in the fridge for 10 min, so the halibut steaks marinade.

3 Bake for 30 minutes to 350°F.
Serve and enjoy!

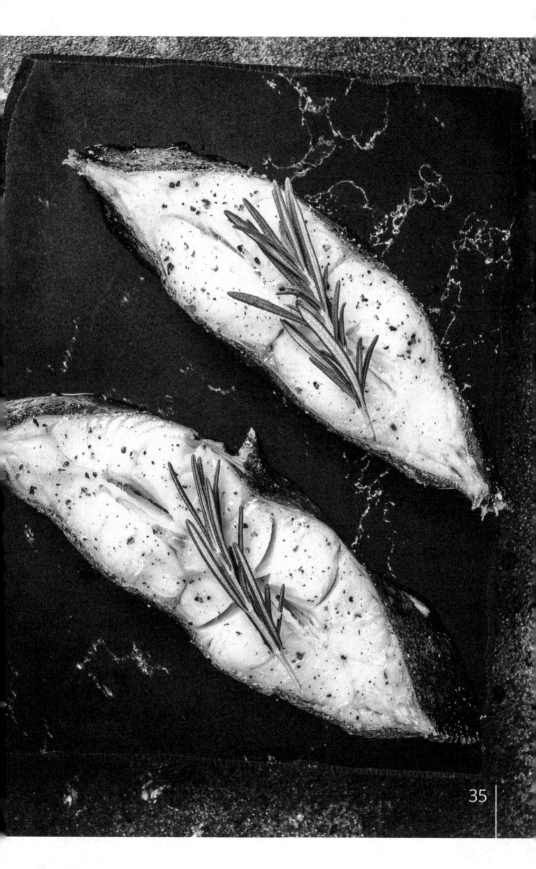

14. Stuffed Artichoke

PREPARATION: 20 MIN

COOKING: 35 MIN

SERVES:6

Ingredients

- 6 whole artichokes
- 3 tablespoons of virgin olive oil
- Salt and pepper
- 2 tablespoons of parsley minced
- 2 boiled potatoes
- 4 tablespoons of Parmesan cheese
- 4 tablespoons of bread crumbs
- 1 egg
- 1 cloves garlic, minced

Directions

1. First of all, with a knife cut off stems of the artichokes.Cut off 1/3 inch of the tips of all of the artichoke leaves. Use a metal spoon to scrape the inner leaves and fuzzy choke.

2. In a bowl, use a fork to mash the potatoes. Then add the parsley, garlic minced, parmesan cheese, one egg, bread crumbs, salt and pepper.
In a pan, place the olive oil with the artichokes and with a teaspoon, fill the artichokes.

3. Cover the pan and cook for 30 minutes to medium heat.
Serve and Enjoy!

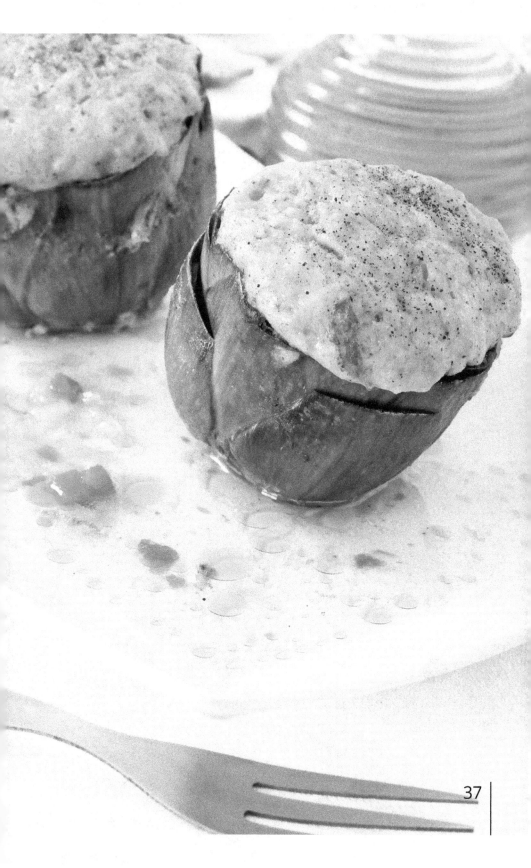

15. Baked Fennels, Red Onion and Olives

 PREPARATION: 5 MIN

 COOKING: 20 MIN

 SERVES:4

Ingredients

- 2 fennels, sliced
- 4 tablespoons of virgin olive oil
- Salt and pepper
- 1 red onion, sliced
- 2 tablespoons of green olives

Directions

1 In a casserole, place the fennels, red onion and green olives. Then mix with olive oil, salt and pepper.

2 Baked for 20 minutes to 350 °F

3 Serve and enjoy!

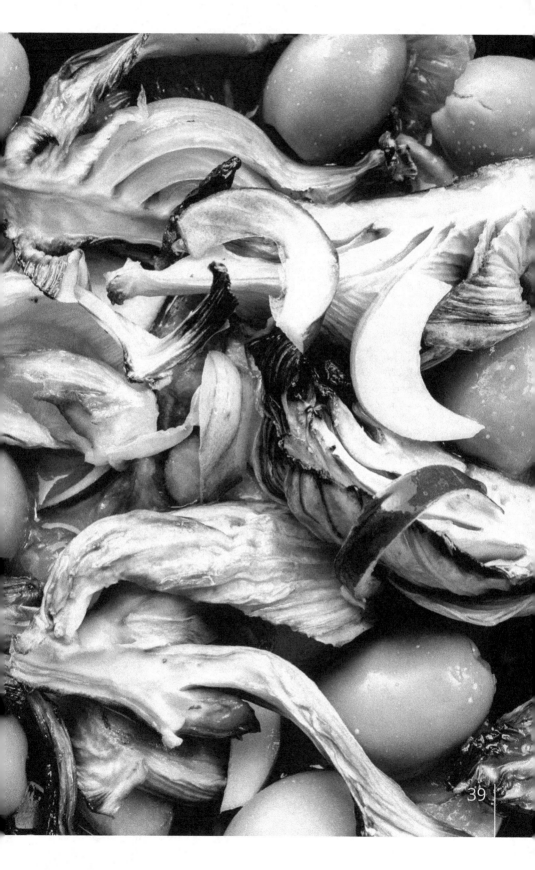

16. Parmigiana Casserole

PREPARATION: 20 MIN

COOKING: 2 h

SERVES: 4

Ingredients

- 4 eggplants
- 1 bottle of tomato puree
- 1 large white onion
- Fresh basil shredded
- Salt and pepper
- Virgin olive oil
- 250 g Parmesan cheese grated

Directions

1. First of all, prepare the tomato sauce: In a pot, put the tomato puree, sliced onion, fresh basil, a pinch of pepper, two teaspoons of salt, two tablespoons of virgin olive oil and mix with a spatula; cook on low heat for 1 hour, check and mix sometimes.

2. Meanwhile, sliced eggplants and grilled. In a casserole, create an eggplants-tomato sauce-parmesan cheese layer until the casserole is filled. Cover and bake to 392°F for 20 minutes, then remove the lid and bake for 40 minutes.

3. Serve and Enjoy!

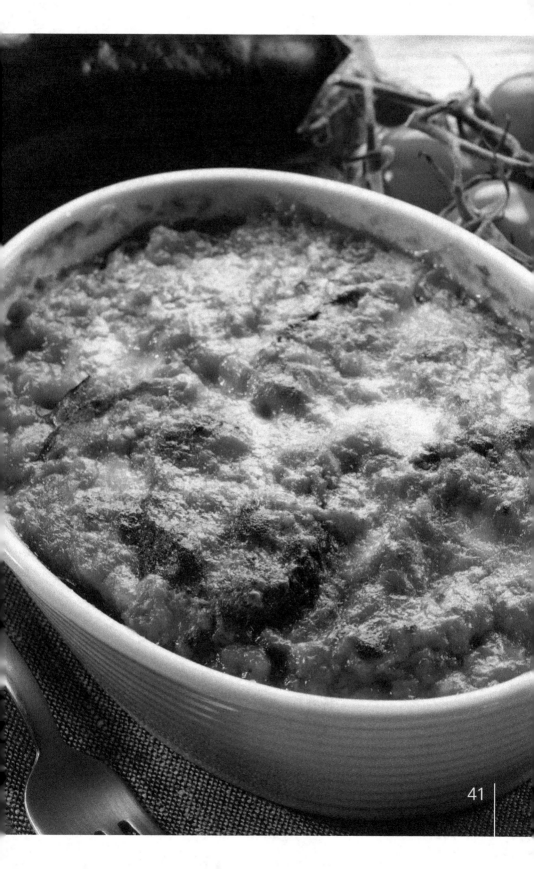

17. Steak Pork Grill With Orange Sauce

PREPARATION: 5 MIN

COOKING: 20 MIN

SERVES: 2

Ingredients

- 2 steaks pork

Orange sauce

- fresh orange juice (from two oranges)
- 2 teaspoon cornstarch
- 2 teaspoon honey
- ½ teaspoon pepper
- ½ teaspoon of cinnamon
- ½ teaspoon salt
- 1/3 cup of white wine

Directions

1 First of all, make the orange sauce: in a saucepan, place orange juice, cornstarch, honey, pepper, cinnamon, salt and white wine. Cook for 8 minutes to low heat until thickened.

2 Grill steaks without condiments.

3 Serve steaks with orange sauce and Enjoy!

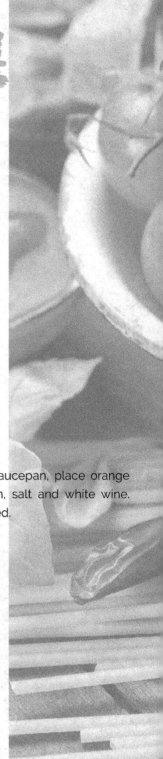

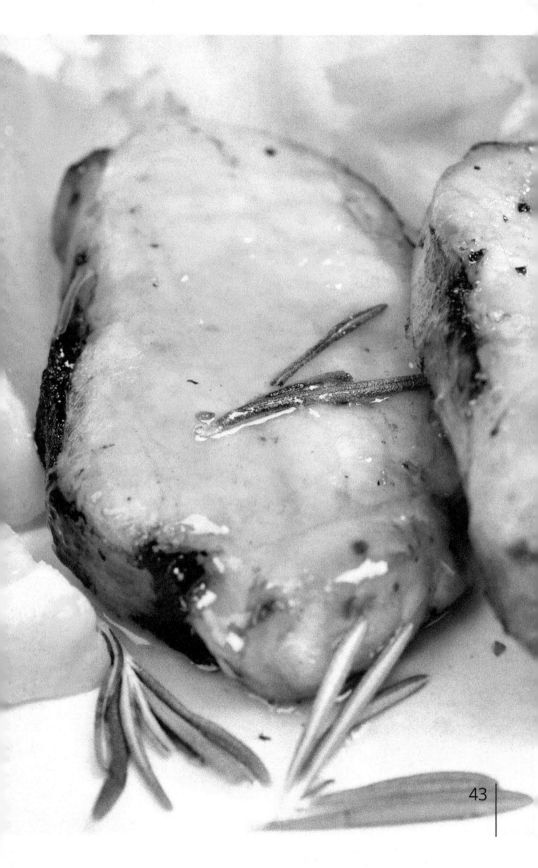

18. Chicken Orange Greek Yogurt Sauce

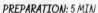

PREPARATION: 5 MIN **COOKING:** 5 MIN **SERVES:** 2

Ingredients

- 250 g chicken strips
- 2 tablespoons Greek yogurt
- 1 orange peeled cubed
- 1 teaspoon pepper
- 1 teaspoon salt
- 1 teaspoon virgin olive oil

Directions

1 In a pan, cook the chicken strips without condiments.

2 In a dish, place the chicken strips and use a fork to mix it with olive oil, salt, pepper, Greek yogurt and orange cubed.

3 Serve and Enjoy!

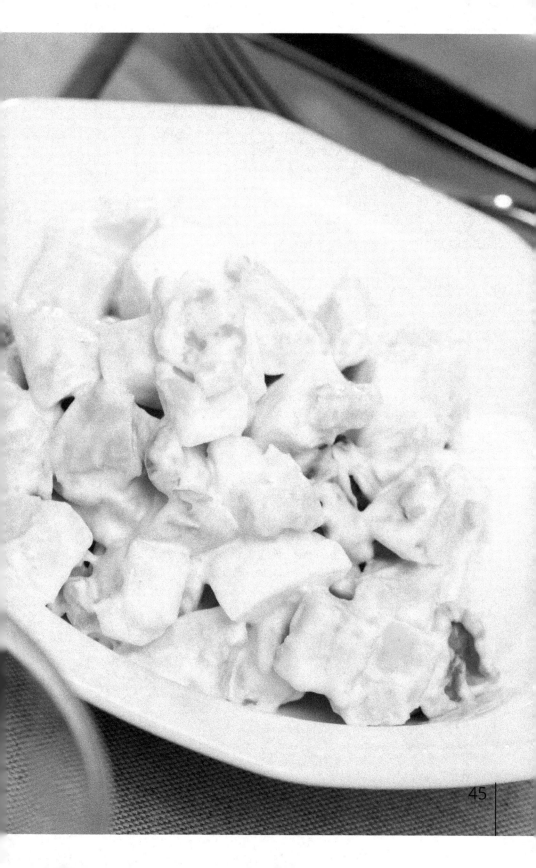

19. Beef Spinach Meatballs

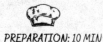 PREPARATION: 10 MIN   COOKING: 25 MIN   SERVES: 2

Ingredients

- 400 g ground beef
- 200 g frozen chopped spinach
- 1 egg
- ½ onion minced
- ½ garlic powder
- 4 tablespoons breadcrumbs
- 2 tablespoons of Parmesan cheese
- 1 teaspoon of pepper
- 1 teaspoon of salt

Directions

1. Preheat your oven to 350°F. In a bowl, combine ground beef, onion, garlic powder, spinach, breadcrumbs, one egg, parmesan cheese, salt and pepper. Form small balls from the mixture and place each ball in a casserole.

2. Bake for 25 minutes per pound at 350 °F.

3. Serve and enjoy!

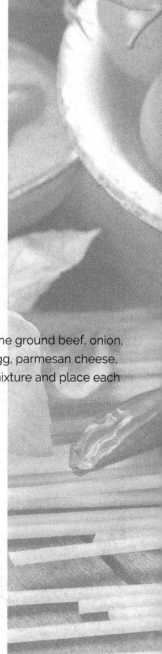

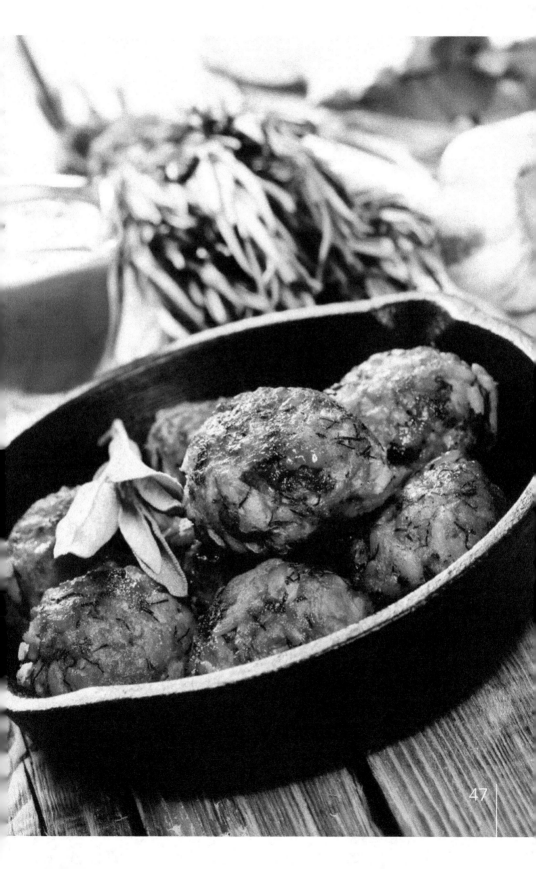

20.Spanish Peas Tortilla

PREPARATION: 25 MIN   COOKING: 20+15 MIN   SERVES: 4

Ingredients

- 6 eggs, whisked
- 4 medium potatoes, peeled and chopped
- 4 tablespoons Parmesan cheese
- 6 tablespoons peas
- 3 tablespoons parsley
- 1 onion chopped
- Salt
- Pepper
- 5 tablespoons virgin olive oil

Directions

1 First of all, cook potatoes and peas: In a pan pour three tablespoons virgin olive oil, potatoes, peas, salt and pepper.
Cover the pan and cook for about 20 minutes to medium heat.

2 Spoon potatoes and peas on a dish allow cooling.
In a bowl, combine six eggs whisked, potatoes, peas, onion, parsley, parmesan cheese, salt, and pepper.

3 In a skillet, heat two tablespoons of virgin olive oil, then add the mixture and cook for about 15 minutes until the sides have golden brown and the tortilla's center baked.
Serve and Enjoy!

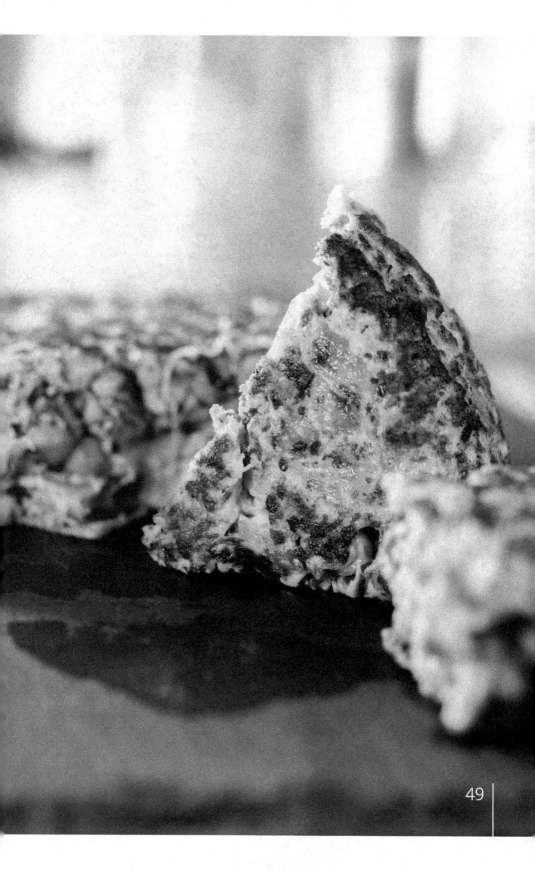

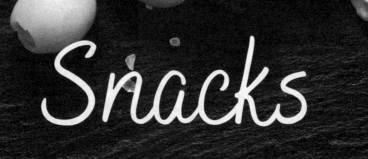

Snacks

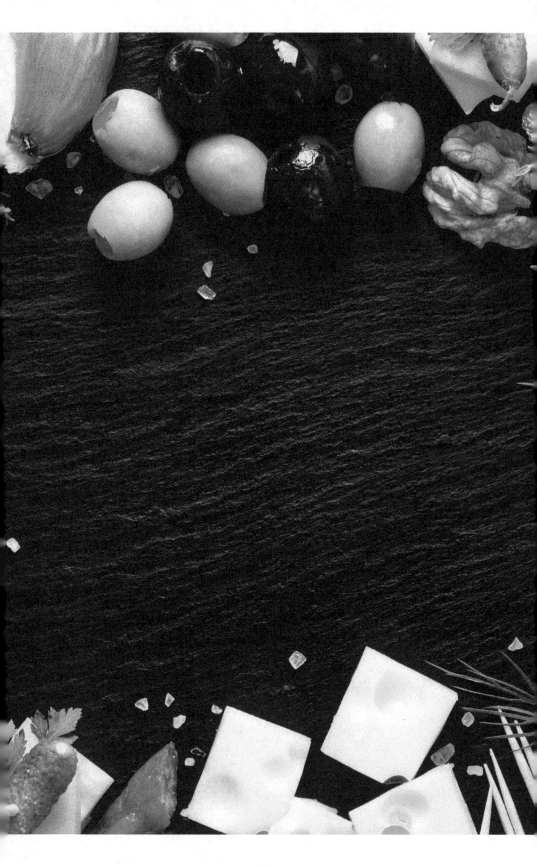

21. Asparagus-Cottage Cheese Cupcake

PREPARATION: 5 MIN

COOKING: 15 min

SERVES: 2

Ingredients

- 250 g cottage cheese
- 2 teaspoons lemon juice
- 1 egg
- 1 teaspoon pepper
- ½ cup asparagus chopped

Directions

1 In a bowl, combine cottage cheese, lemon juice, one egg, pepper and asparagus.

2 Mix all ingredients with a silicone spoon, then pour the mixture into muffin cups. Bake for 15 minutes to 350˚F.

3 Serve and Enjoy!

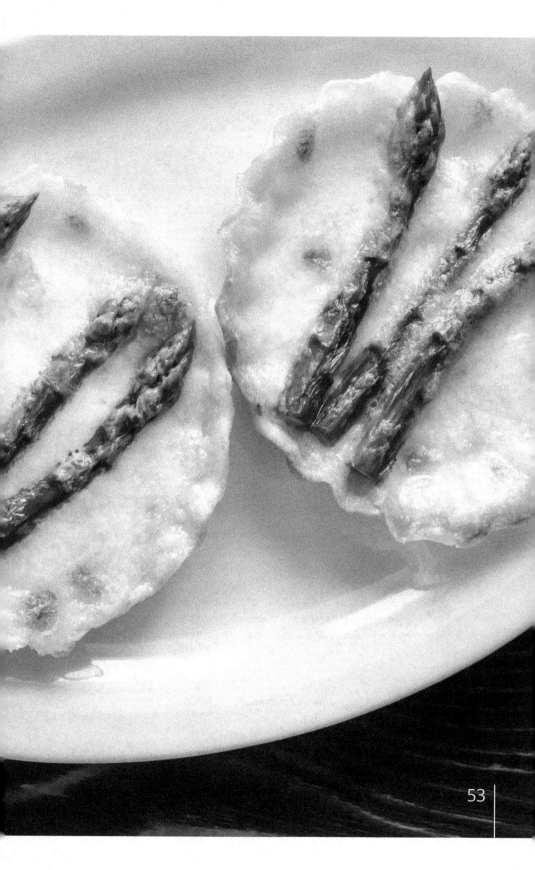

22. Raw Ham Stuffed Boiled Eggs

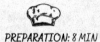
PREPARATION: 8 MIN

COOKING: 6 min

SERVES: 4

Ingredients

- 8 eggs
- 1 teaspoon mustard
- 2 tablespoons mayonnaise
- 2 tablespoons raw ham cubed
- 1 teaspoon pepper
- 1 teaspoon lemon juice
- Capers, for garnish

Directions

1 In a saucepan, place the eggs, cover them with water. Bring just to a boil for 3 minutes.

2 Spoon eggs on a dish allow cooling. Peel eggs and slice in half, Remove yolks and place in a small bowl with the ingredients: raw ham, mayonnaise, mustard, lemon juice, and pepper. Mix until creamy.

3 Top each egg white half with about 1 ½ teaspoon mixture.
If desired, garnish with capers.
Serve and Enjoy!

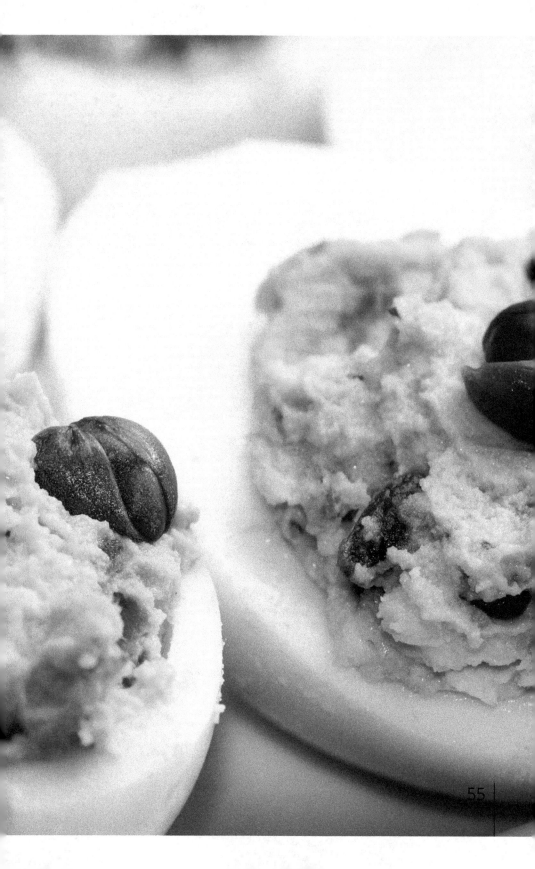

23. Carrot-Cucumber Creamy

PREPARATION: 5 MIN

COOKING: 0 MIN

SERVES: 1

Ingredients

- ½ cucumber, peeled and chopped
- 2 tablespoons Greek yogurt
- 1 tablespoon cream cheese
- 2 teaspoons lemon juice
- ½ carrot chopped
- Pinch of salt
- 1 teaspoon chives chopped
- Fresh vegetables, for serving

Directions

1 In a bowl, place carrot, cucumber, a pinch of salt, lemon juice, and chives.

2 Then add Greek yogurt, cream cheese, and with a wooden spoon, combine all ingredient until creamy.

3 Serve with fresh vegetables and enjoy!

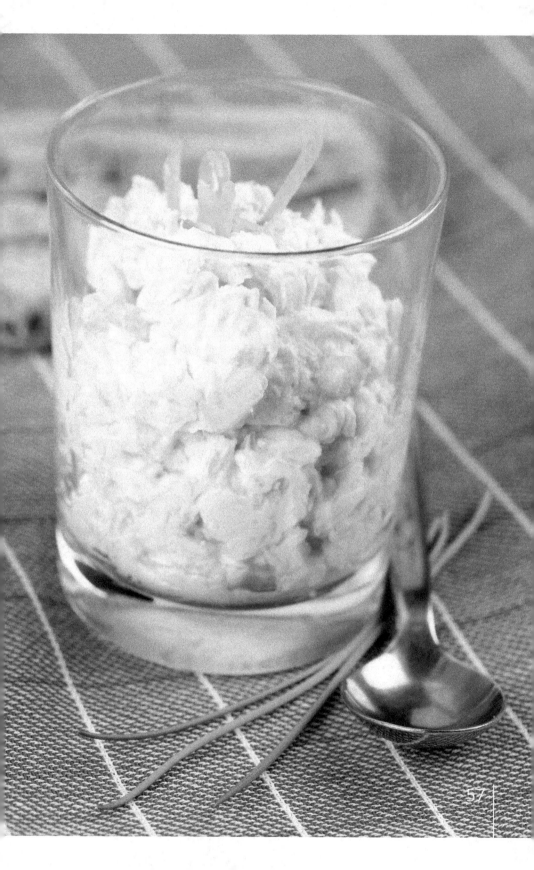

24. Grill Zucchini– Smoked Salmon Rolls

 PREPARATION: 5 MIN

 COOKING: 6 min.

 SERVES: 1

Ingredients

- 5 slices long side zucchini to roll
- Salt
- 5 slices smoked salmon
- 5 toothpicks

Directions

1 First of all, preheat your grill to medium heat. Then grill the zucchini slices for about 3 minutes on each side.

2 In a dish place, the zucchini allow cooling. Then salt it and roll each zucchini slice with smoked salmon slices. Secure the roll with a toothpick.

3 Serve and Enjoy!

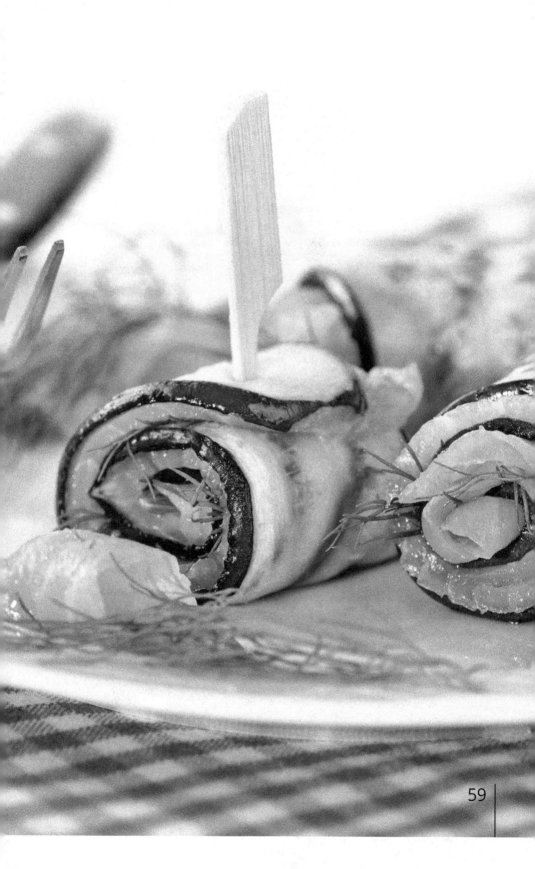

25. Italian Three Color Frittata

PREPARATION: 10 MIN

COOKING: 25 MIN

SERVES: 4

Ingredients

- 6 dried cherry tomatoes, sliced
- 2 eggs, whisked
- 2 tablespoons of Feta cheese
- 6 fresh basil leaves
- 1 tablespoon unsalted butter
- Salt and pepper

Directions

1. In an 8-inch nonstick skillet, melt the butter over low heat.
   In a small bowl, whisk eggs and add salt and pepper. Then pour all in the skillet and cook for about 2 minutes on each side until golden. Use a silicone spatula to turn the frittata on both sides.

2. Fill the frittata with feta, basil, and tomatoes. Fold it in half and serve!

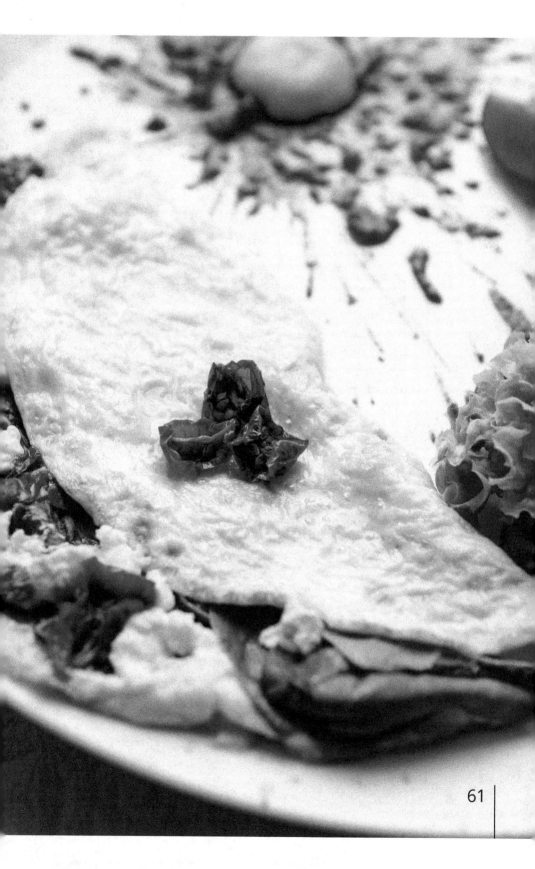

26. Tuna Creamy

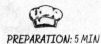

PREPARATION: 5 MIN   COOKING: 0 MIN   SERVES: 1

Ingredients

- 1 canned tuna
- 1 teaspoon capers
- 1 teaspoon lemon juice
- 2 tablespoon mayonnaise
- Pita chips, for serving

Directions

1 In a blender, combine tuna, lemon juice, capers and mayonnaise until they reach the desired consistency.

2 Serve with pita chips and enjoy!

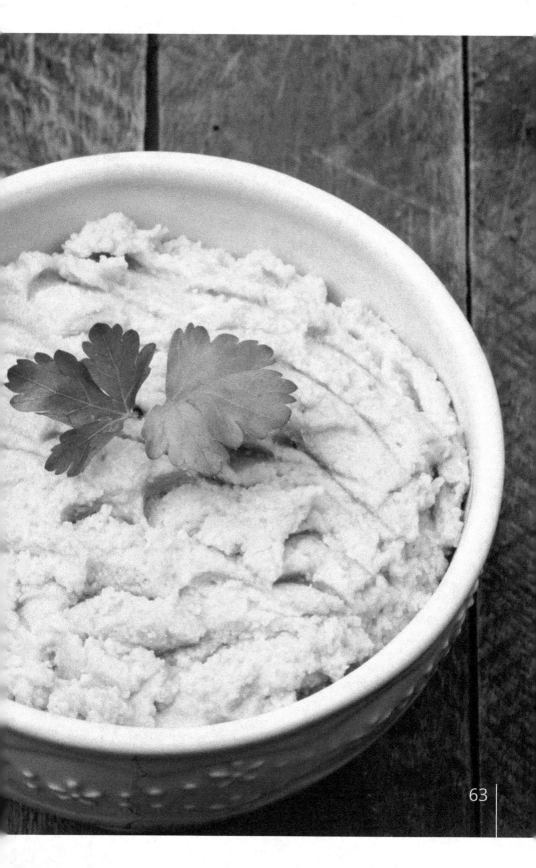

27. Fried Zucchini With Fresh Tomatoes and Cream Cheese

PREPARATION: 5 MIN

COOKING: 5 MIN

SERVES: 2

Ingredients

- 2 tablespoons virgin olive oil
- 1 zucchini, sliced
- 1 small fresh tomato, sliced
- low-fat cream cheese

Directions

1. In a pot, pour two tablespoons of virgin olive oil and heat for 2 minutes. Then add the zucchini slices and fry for 5 minutes per side.

2. In a dish, place the fried zucchini; on each slice, spread ½ teaspoon cream cheese and add one tomato slice.

3. Serve and Enjoy!

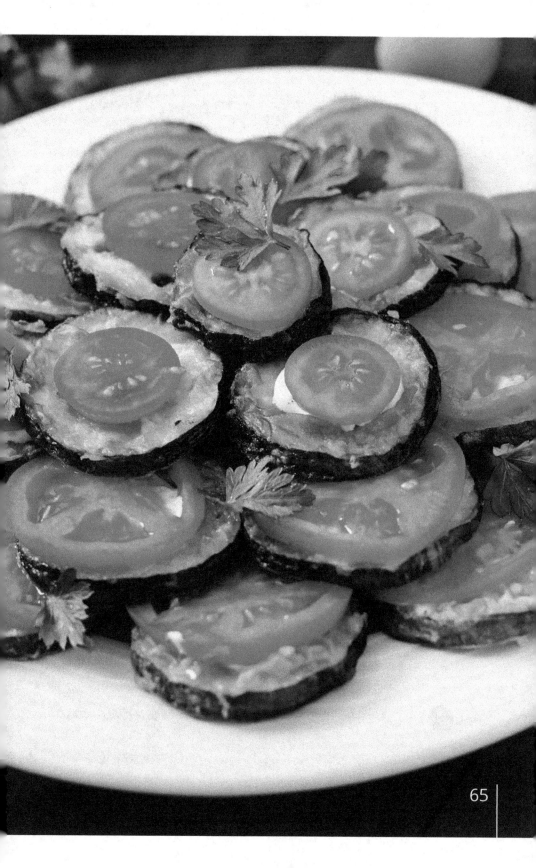

28. Cherry Tomatoes Baked

PREPARATION: 5 MIN

COOKING: 20 min

SERVES: 4

Ingredients

- 20 cherry tomatoes, halved
- Virgin olive oil
- Salt and pepper
- 3 teaspoons of oregano

Directions

1 In a casserole, place the cherry tomatoes halved, salt and pepper, and sprinkle the cherry tomatoes with olive oil and oregano.

2 Baked for 20 minutes to 350 °F.

3 Serve and Enjoy!

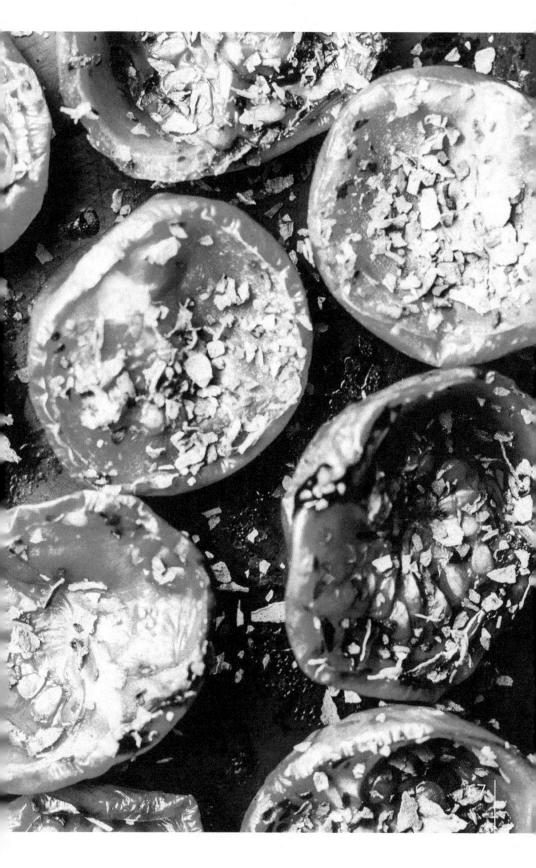

29.Baked Cauliflower Spicy

 PREPARATION: 5 MIN   **COOKING:** 20 MIN   **SERVES:** 4

Ingredients

- 1 teaspoon of paprika
- ½ teaspoon of garlic powder
- ½ teaspoon of black pepper
- 4 heads cauliflower
- 4 tablespoons of virgin olive oil
- 1 ½ teaspoon of pink salt
- 2 teaspoon parsley, chopped

Directions

1 Mix paprika, garlic powder, black pepper, pink salt, and virgin olive oil in a bowl. For each head cauliflower sides, evenly sprinkle the mixture and then place in a casserole.

2 Cover the casserole with foil and bake for 10 minutes to 392˚F.
Remove the foil, flip the cauliflowers, and roast for 10 minutes until brown crust forms.

3 Serve with parsley and Enjoy!

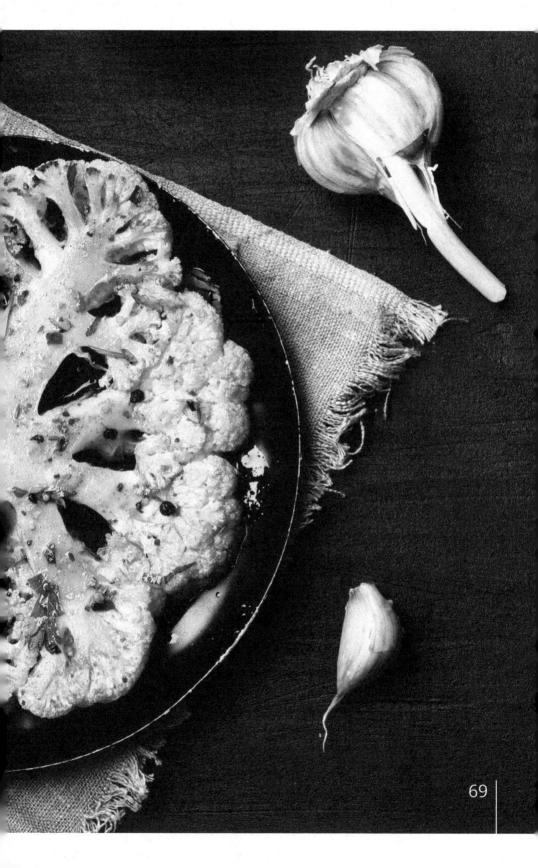

30. Black Olive Creamy Paté

PREPARATION: 10 MIN

COOKING: 0 MIN

SERVES: 2

Ingredients

- ½ cup pitted black olives
- 2 tablespoons virgin olive oil
- 1 teaspoon lemon juice
- 1 teaspoon capers
- ½ teaspoon dried rosemary
- toasted bread, for serving

Directions

1 In a blender, combine black olives, lemon juice, capers, virgin olive oil, rosemary and blend until creamy.

2 Serve with toast bread and enjoy!

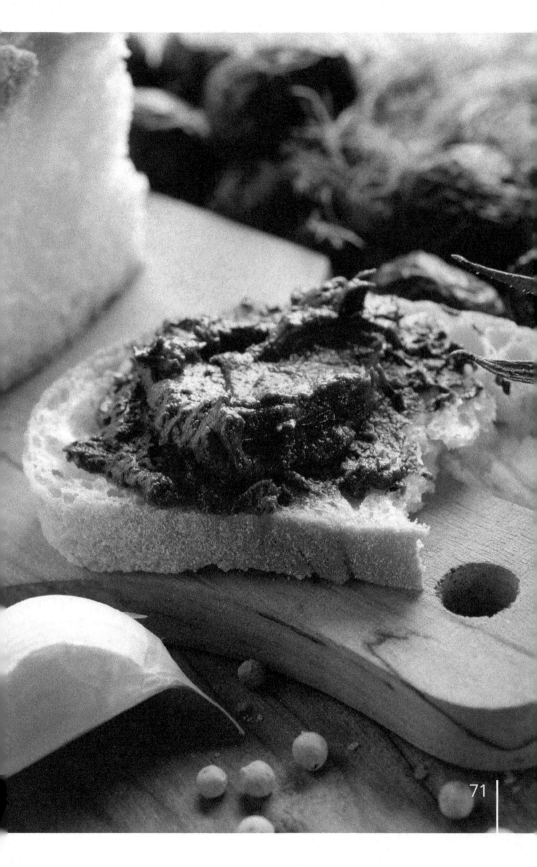

Dinner

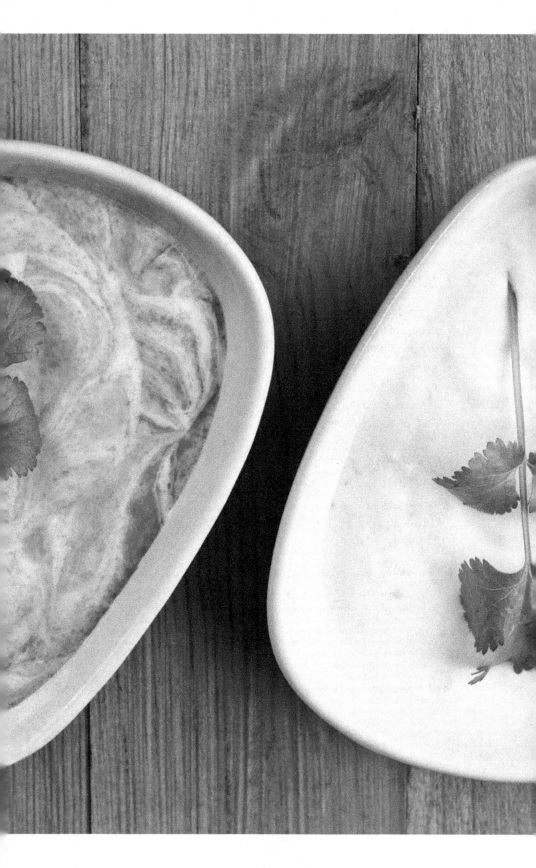

31. Tuna Olives Pasta

PREPARATION: 5 MIN

COOKING: 10 min

SERVES: 2

Ingredients

- 1 cup dry fusilli pasta
- ½ cup of fresh tuna, diced
- ½ cup of black olives
- 5 cherry tomatoes chopped
- 1 ½ tablespoon of olive oil
- ½ teaspoon of salt
- Salt for cook the pasta

Directions

1 **Pasta sauce**
In a skillet, cook tuna with olive oil, cherry tomatoes, black olives for 6-7 minutes.

2 Meanwhile, cook the pasta: take the pot, fill with water, and bring it to a boil. Pour the salt into the boiling water. When the salt is dissolved, put the pasta and cook as instructed.

3 Mix pasta with pasta sauce and serve.

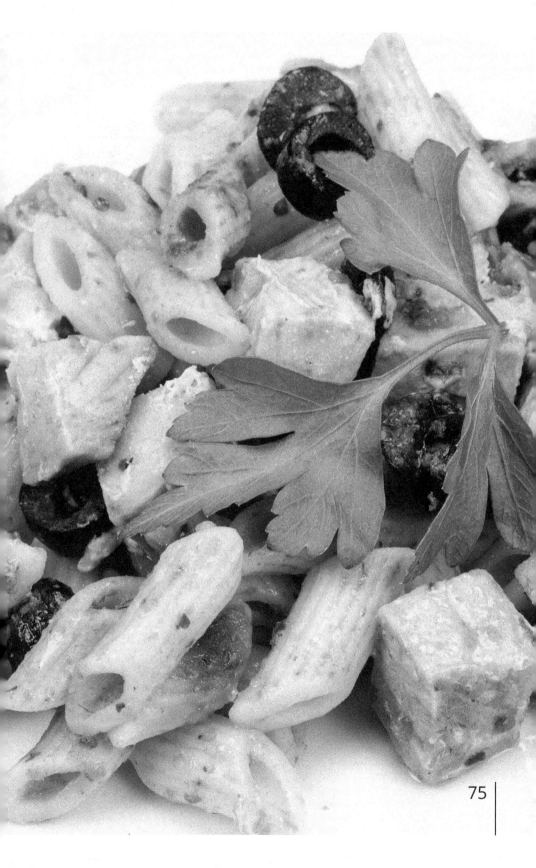

32. Asparagus Cream Soup

PREPARATION: 10 MIN

COOKING: 30 min

SERVES: 4

Ingredients

- 20 diced asparagus
- 1 chopped onion
- 1 L of vegetable stock
- 2 tablespoons of Virgin olive oil
- 1 potato sliced
- ½ teaspoon pepper

Directions

1 In a pot, sautè of onion for 5 minutes; then add asparagus and potato and mix. Add the vegetable stock and cook for 30 minutes.

2 Use the hand-held blender to mix and serve.

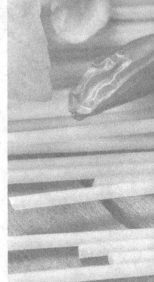

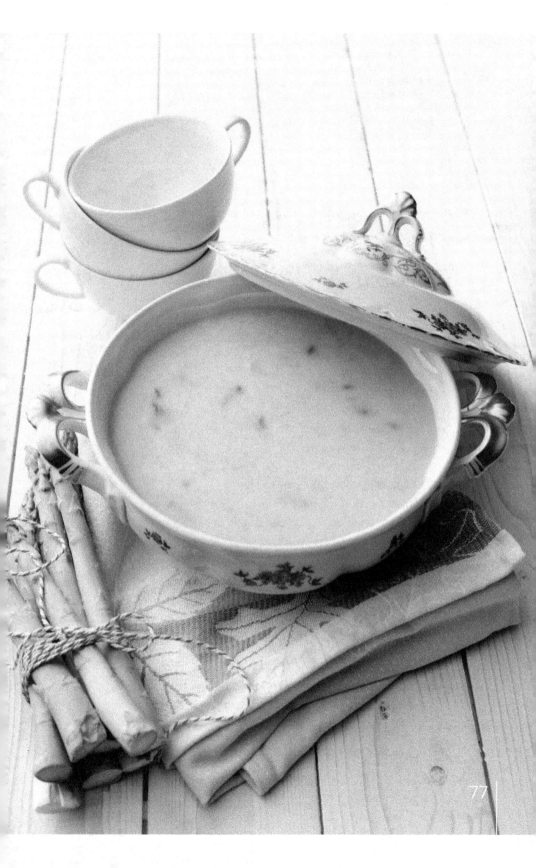

33. Fish Soup

PREPARATION: 10 MIN

COOKING: 55 min

SERVES: 1

Ingredients

- 1 bottle of tomato puree
- 4 cups of water
- 3 tablespoons powder vegetable stock
- 1 cod fillet, diced
- 10 prawns
- ½ kg of mussels
- 3 tablespoons chopped parsley
- ¼ teaspoon chili pepper
- 1 carrot sliced
- 2 cloves of garlic, chopped
- 3 tablespoons Virgin olive oil
- 3 tablespoon chopped celery

Directions

1. First of all, clean and wash the mussels. In a pot, put the olive oil and the garlic sauté for 5 minutes. Add the mussels, prawns, cod fillet and mix for 1 minute.

2. Add the carrot, vegetable stock, celery, chili pepper, tomato puree, parsley, and water; cover the pot and cook for 50 minutes.

3. Serve and Enjoy!

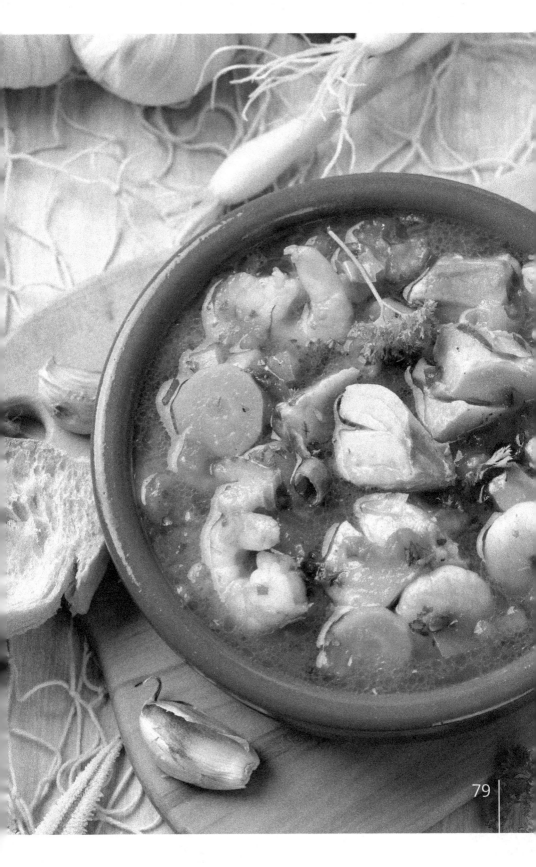

34. Pumpkin Soup

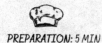
PREPARATION: 5 MIN

COOKING: 30 MIN

SERVES: 4

Ingredients

- ½ cup tahini
- Pinch of salt
- ¼ cup virgin olive oil
- ¼ cup warm water
- 1 teaspoon lemon juice
- ½ clove garlic, minced

Directions

1 In a pot, put the water and all ingredients and cook for 30 minutes. Then turn off the pot and mix with a hand-held blender.

2 It is ready, serve and enjoy!

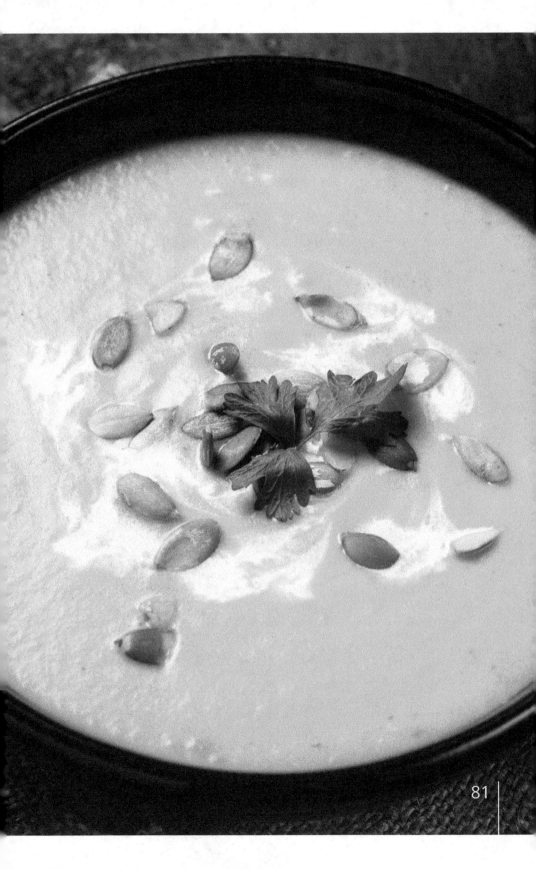

35.Beans Soup

PREPARATION: 10 MIN   COOKING: 30 min   SERVES: 4

Ingredients

- 500 g of beans
- 1 onion
- 2 tomatoes
- 2 carrots
- ½ celery
- 4 tablespoons virgin olive oil
- Salt and pepper to taste
- 1L water

Directions

1   Chop the following ingredients: onion, carrots, and celery. Then slice the tomatoes.

2   In a pot, put the cold water and all ingredients and cook for 30 minutes.
Serve hot and enjoy!

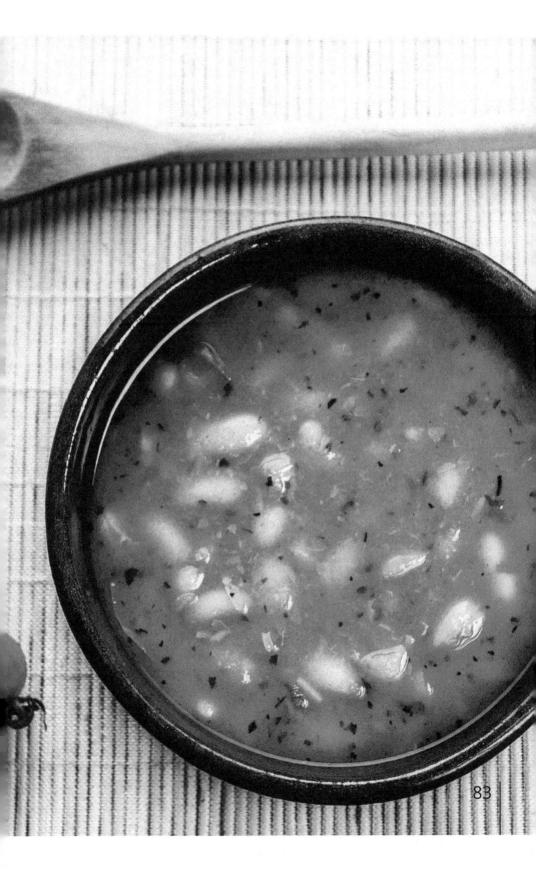

36. Minestrone Green Soup

PREPARATION: 5 MIN

COOKING:1 0/40 MIN

SERVES: 4

Ingredients

- 4 chopped courgettes
- 1 onion chopped
- 2 carrots chopped
- 1 potato chopped
- 1 cup of broccoli chopped
- 2 tablespoons powder vegetable stock
- 500 ml water

Directions

1 In a pressure cooker, put all ingredients and mix and cook for 10 minutes.

2 If you don't have a pressure cooker, use a normal pot and cook for 40 minutes.

3 Serve and Enjoy!

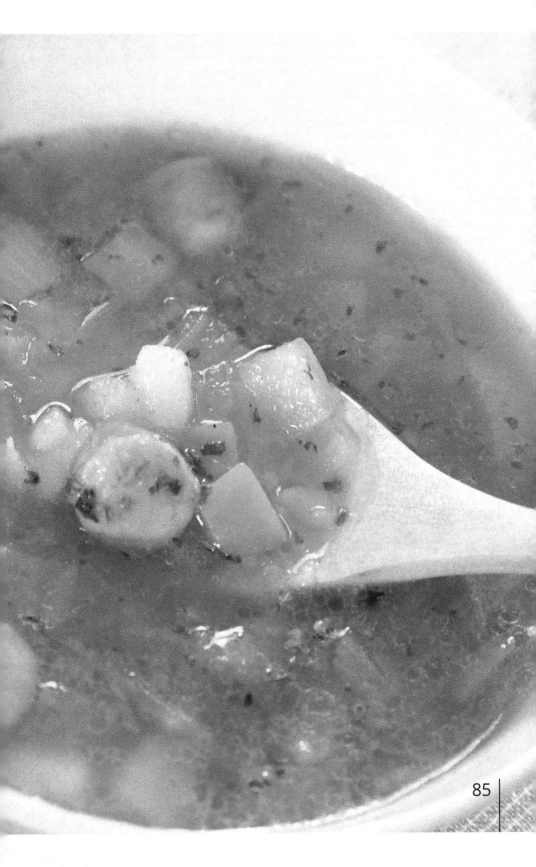

37. Saffron Risotto

PREPARATION: 20 MIN

COOKING: 40 min

SERVES: 4

Ingredients

- ¼ teaspoon of saffron
- 600 ml vegetable stock
- ½ chopped onion
- Virgin olive oil
- 1 teaspoon of butter
- Parmesan cheese for garnish
- 350 g rice

Directions

1 First of all, heat the vegetable stock. In a pot, sauté the onion for 7-8 minutes. Then put the rice and mix with a wooden spoon.

2 Add some vegetable stock until cover all rice and mix. (When the rice has absorbed all the stock, add the vegetable stock again.) repeat this process two times until rice is almost cooked.

3 When the rice is almost cooked, add the saffron and butter and mix for 1 minute.
Serve with Parmesan cheese and Enjoy!

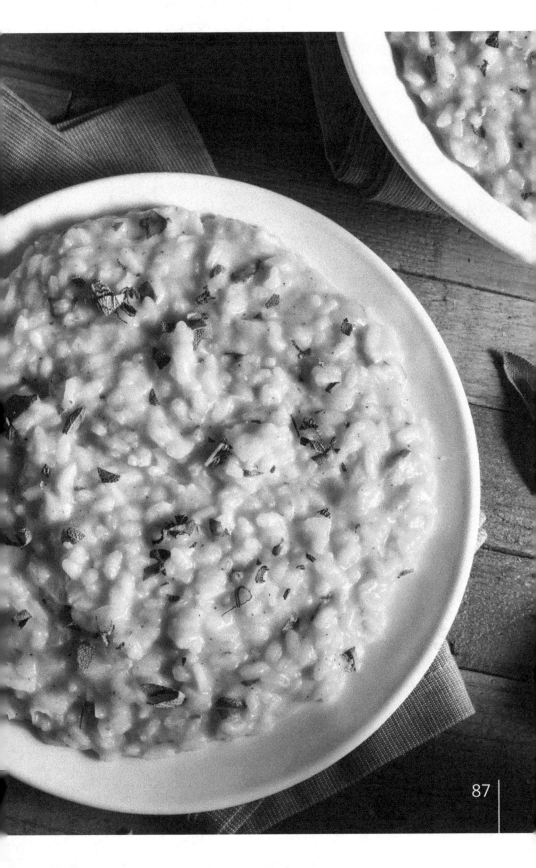

38. Herb Baked Fillets Tuna

PREPARATION: 10 MIN

COOKING: 0 MIN

SERVES: 4

Ingredients

- 2 tuna fillets
- 2 teaspoons of lemon juice
- 2 tablespoons of olive oil
- 1 teaspoon of salt
- 1 teaspoon of pepper
- 1 teaspoon of oregano
- 1 teaspoon of thyme
- 1 teaspoon of garlic powder
- 1 teaspoon of dried basil
- 1 teaspoon of rosemary

Directions

1. In a resealable plastic bag, put the olive oil, lemon juice, garlic powder, and all spices.

2. Add tuna fillets and rub the seasonings. Seal the bag and put it in the fridge for 20 min, so the tuna fillets marinade.

3. In a little casserole, place the tuna fillets and bake for 15-20 minutes to 350°F.
Serve and enjoy!

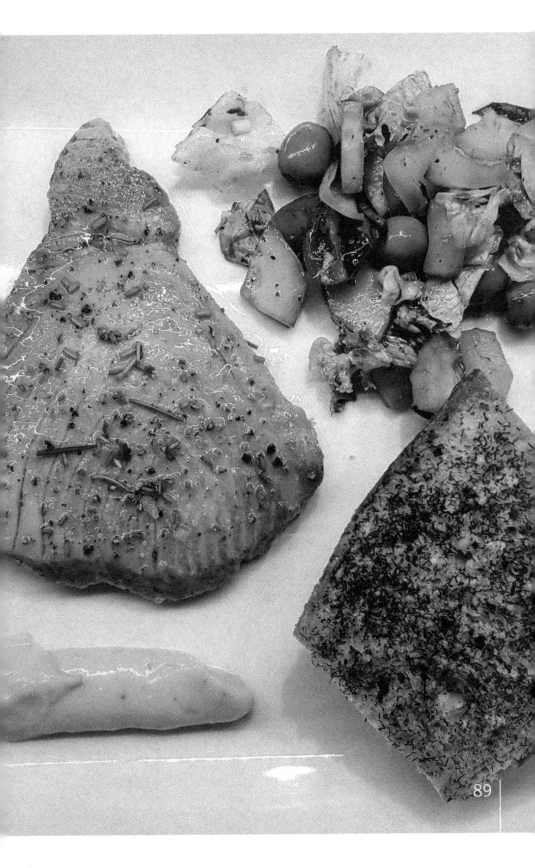

39. Shrimps in Tomato-Parsley Sauce

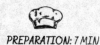
PREPARATION: 7 MIN

COOKING: 30 min

SERVES: 3

Ingredients

- 3 tablespoons of parsley
- 1 pinch of chili pepper
- 1 onion, chopped
- 2 teaspoons of pepper
- 400 g of shrimps
- 2 tablespoons of olive oil
- 300 g of tomato sauce

Directions

1 First of all, in a pot, put the olive oil sauté the chopped onions.

2 Add the missing ingredients, stir and cover the pot for 30 minutes.

3 Serve with bread and enjoy!

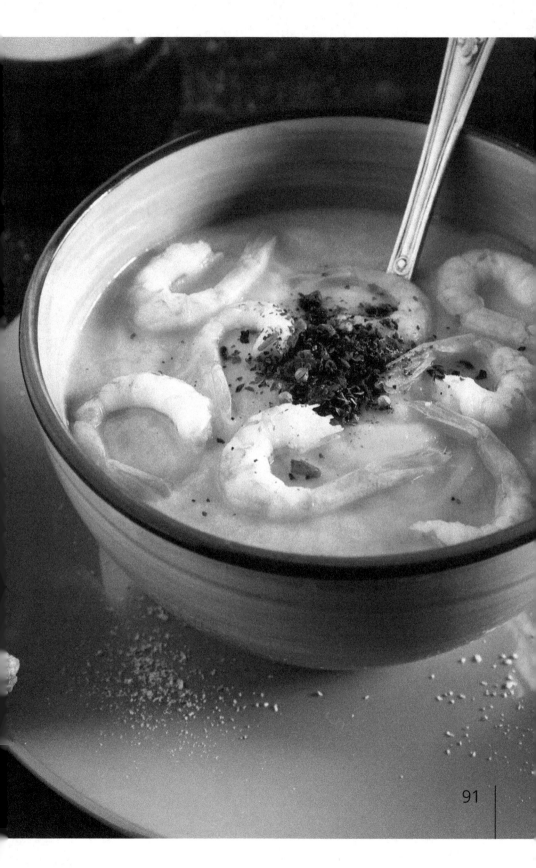

40. Vegetable Turkey Couscous

PREPARATION: 5 MIN

COOKING: 20 min

SERVES: 4

Ingredients

- 1 eggplant chopped
- 2 little peppers chopped
- 1 onion chopped
- 200 ml vegetable broth
- 1 teaspoon curry
- Salt and pepper
- 200 g Couscous
- 300 g turkey meat, diced

Directions

1 In a pan, put the olive oil, eggplant, onion, peppers chopped, one teaspoon of curry, meat, salt, and pepper. Mix all ingredients and cook for 15 minutes to medium heat.

2 Then add couscous and vegetable broth, cover the pan and cook until the couscous has soaked up all the vegetable broth (for about 5-7 minutes).

3 Serve with bread and enjoy!

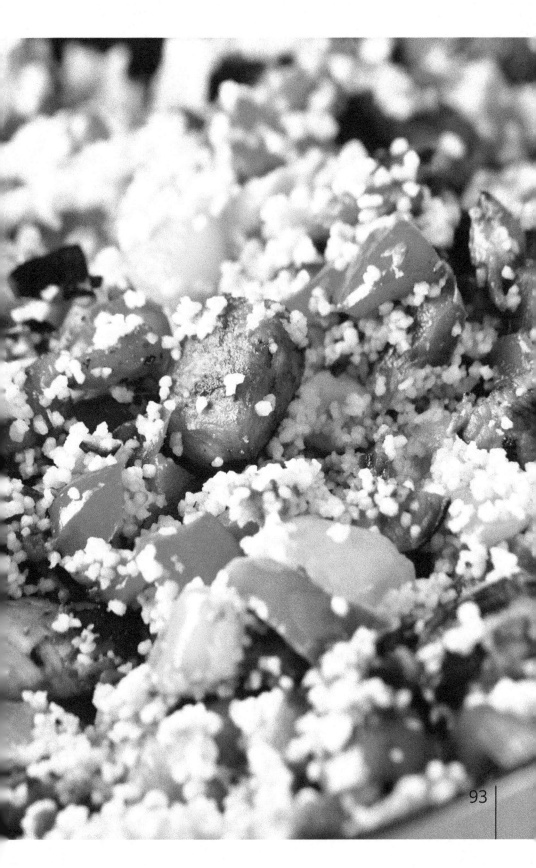